Be *the* CEO *of*
Your Own Health

Be *the* CEO *of* Your Own Health

Create Your Perfect, Feel-Good Lifestyle

Maria Teresa Kline

NEW YORK

LONDON • NASHVILLE • MELBOURNE • VANCOUVER

Be *the* CEO *of* Your Own Health
Create Your Perfect, Feel-Good Lifestyle

© 2020 Maria Teresa Kline

Published in New York, New York, by Morgan James Publishing in partnership with Difference Press. Morgan James is a trademark of Morgan James, LLC. www.MorganJamesPublishing.com

ISBN 978-1-64279-575-2 paperback
ISBN 978-1-64279-576-9 eBook
ISBN 978-1-64279-577-6 Audio
Library of Congress Control Number: 2019939276:

Cover Design by:
Rachel Lopez
www.r2cdesign.com

Interior Design by:
Bonnie Bushman
The Whole Caboodle Graphic Design

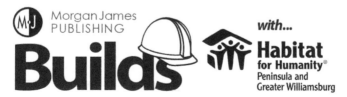

Morgan James is a proud partner of Habitat for Humanity Peninsula and Greater Williamsburg. Partners in building since 2006.

Get involved today! Visit
www.MorganJamesBuilds.com

This book is dedicated to:

My wonderful daughters, you bring me joy.
My mom and dad for everything.
My teachers for their service to humanity.

Table of Contents

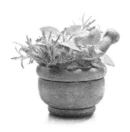

Chapter 1

Facing the Future of Your Health

I write this book for those that have worked hard their whole lives to be successful financially and offer something to the world as well as to themselves and their family. If this is you, then I am talking to you. To be driven in such a way that leaves you at the top of whatever empire you have built is phenomenal. Maybe childhood insecurities have been the driving force behind your success. Maybe fears of not being able to have the financial freedom that your parents had are behind your motivation and success. Maybe the opposite is true, being tired of not having enough growing up was your motivation. Either way, what you need now is the ability to live a long and active life around your present financial success. It does no good to wish and hope for an escape from the voluminous onset of autoimmune diseases besetting our populations at this current time in our lives! Speaking of these problems is not designed to instill fear in anyone, rather to point out that even though we are under a barrage of illnesses in our country, it is important to face these conditions around us and not to look away, burying our heads in the sand. We must not look away. Fearing the doctor is understandable, but avoiding certain knowledge of our health is not! Our country has been changed from what at one point was considered the leading nation in health care to one of the least successful. The United States ranks thirty-seventh on the list of the world's health systems according to the World Health Organization (WHO). We now have more autoimmune diseases than ever before. Some physicians and healers even classify cancer as an autoimmune disease because it attacks us from within…and it is rampant! How did this happen?

From the Land of the Free to the Land of So Many Illnesses
To understand why there is confusion about what is good for you and what is not, we must first look at what is driving the information we get. The medical profession has changed drastically. There was a time when doctors made house calls. This might seem crazy in today's world, but it is true. Now a doctor is very unlikely to make a house call unless he/she is handsomely paid for this "extra" service, or unless the patient is a very good friend to the doctor. Today a doctor with his own practice is heavily burdened by malpractice insurance and the terms of his profession dictated by the government, among other reasons. Doctors today can't spend more than the required time set for all of the patients he sees in a day, which limits the amount of information he is provided with. Essentially, doctors work long hours and have little time to think sideways when it comes to personal attention for any of his or her patients. A doctor in this country also has very little nutritional education in his curriculum at med school, including pre-med. This makes for a difficult situation for most of us. How are we to trust our doctor when he/she is looking through the same lens he does for everyone else? He has no choice. His hands are tied. A doctor in this country can only legally treat a person with

cancer in three ways, with surgery, radiation therapy, and/or chemotherapy. Yes, if a doctor or any healer makes a claim that they can cure anything by any other means, or protocol involving anything other than these three methods, they are subject to warnings, fines and ultimately arrests. A famous case of this in action is that of Dr. Andrew Weil, MD. He is a well-known professor at the medical school in Tucson, AZ. He has become known for his teachings using nutrition to support health, and is widely respected. Yet the FDA and the FTC warned him that if he did not stop suggesting that improving your immune system would help prevent you from getting the flu, he would be fined and sent to jail. His situation was well documented in the media. This example provided shows how difficult it can be for the majority of us to figure out what to believe and how to proceed living out a healthy and happy life in a country where there is so much intended confusion around health.

Nutrition Is Key to Understanding the Causes of Illness
Health problems will still remain if only the symptoms are treated.

The industry held responsible for making medicine to heal us has been accused, according to many news sources today, of defrauding the population, finding that big pharma is only interested in profits. The regulation of these entities is questionable at best and now their intentions are being questioned. Are pharmaceutical companies really making the best medicines to cure us of our maladies as a population? Or are they looking to make a profit? As an American, I would say both. I would have to stipulate that while pharmaceutical companies are in the business to make medicine, I do not think that their medicine is for cures anymore, but for symptoms. Just like putting a band aid on a cut. You are only treating the symptom, or what you can see. You are not treating the cause. You are not making an attempt at stopping the problem. No one is giving you instructions on how to change something, or take something, that will get rid of your problem. Only to relieve the symptoms of your problem. This does not sound like a solution, does it? It seems like once you have been prescribed a heart medicine or something for high blood pressure, it is a life sentence. Wouldn't you feel better knowing that you were doing something to get rid of the problem forever and be well again? Taking a pharmaceutical drug has its consequences, they are called side effects. Sometimes these side effects outweigh the original problem.

Listening to a television commercial advertise a new drug that has come out and hearing that a possible side effect is sudden death can't feel right!

Symptomatic treatment is the existing paradigm of our health care system that dominates today. We are training professionals to treat our symptoms, not the cause. Perhaps it is because we still cannot agree on the causes of things. If you are reading this book, it might mean that you have lost faith in the existing model of health care that is current in our country. A new model has been appearing all over and has taken hold in many areas of our culture. Alternative medicine is the general term for what is considered the alternative to allopathic medicine, which is sanctioned by our system. The word alternative suggests a choice. I like choices. We all have to learn to make a choice for ourselves based on what we believe to be true and righteous. In order to make a choice we must be informed. I believe that is why you are reading this book.

"Physician, heal thyself!"—Aeschylus circa 525/524 BCE
Becoming the CEO of your own health is a reality. You do not need a medical degree to understand how you feel and what your particular system needs to feel better. I admit

that for a broken bone or some such problem, a physician is exactly whom I would see. It is a relief to know that we have hospitals and ambulances for the sick. The problem we face is how to understand the term "sick." We can be sick long before heading to the hospital with symptoms we've ignored through fear. This is one of the dangers we need to address as a society. We must all understand that when a doctor determines that you have cancer, you have most likely had this in your body for ten years at least. When my mother was diagnosed with cancer, that is exactly what the physician told me.

I have also realized that one cancer patient is worth a very large amount of money for the duration of the illness. It is much more difficult to play the "catch up" game than it is to nip something in the bud. The first thing we must face is the word cancer. There is no greater devastation than to go to the doctor for a persistent headache and be told you have stage 4 cancer. This was my mother's case. If you have been living a productive life, headaches notwithstanding, and you receive this diagnosis from a medical professional, I can assure you that you might lose all hope. It becomes a testament to one's character to be strong enough to stand up to that diagnosis and continue to live a meaningful life, however long you may have. This is not what we want to struggle with. We want to have choices. We want to understand how to fight, and how to feel better, eliminating the fear from our lives. The first big step is education. By reading this book you have taken the first step to finding out what kind of choices are available to us. We all have the ability to reverse our biological age if we so choose. How do we do that? The answer is not complicated but it does take time to begin to shift that paradigm we have been programmed to believe since our birth. Science and technology have advanced faster in these last few decades than ever before in our human history. The study of genetics has uncovered many things that we were unaware of previously. The most important fact we must understand is that genetics can be turned off as much as it can be turned on. This means that if your grandmother or someone in your immediate family died of cancer, it does not necessarily mean that you will get cancer. There have been many studies done on cancer.

In a landmark study, published in the *Journal of the National Cancer Institute* in 1981, it was found that U.S. cancer deaths could be reduced by 90% for stomach and large bowel cancers: 50% for breast cancer, uterus, gallbladder, and pancreatic cancers; 20 % for larynx, bladder, cervix, mouth pharynx, and esophagus cancers; and 10 % for other cancers. The study commissioned by the U.S. Congress wanted to determine the extent to which cancer is avoidable. The conclusion was that tobacco and diet were the biggest cancer-causing culprits. Yes, diet is at the top of the list. What is being understood at this point in our evolution is that a lifestyle change is necessary for us to live out our lives in peace and health. So much of our advertising goes to food. We are urged to eat every few minutes with every commercial we endure to get to the end of our show. We are seduced by a barrage of images of food while we drive, while we watch TV, and while we peruse the internet or play with our phones. It is almost too much to resist. Resist we must, and reading this book is a way to better understand your risks and to learn how to reduce your own chances of developing autoimmune diseases and even cancer.

Given that diet is at the forefront in the fight for our lives, we are called to study the effects and the truths of food. We must also shed some light on the kind of lifestyle that will both bring happiness and a wealth of health to our lives. Only then can we be confident in our everyday choices and live out a life of peaceful bliss with those around us. You have worked hard to enjoy the finer things in life, now find the space to bring this same focus to your new health lifestyle.

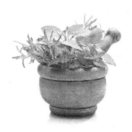

Chapter 2

Owning My Health and Nutrition

Growing up I traveled a ton. I was literally exposed to probably every disease known to man. I exaggerate. But not by much. I grew up on five of the seven continents. I was vaccinated against everything that had an existing vaccine, and some that didn't. My parents were very healthy people according to most modern standards. They had never been sick as long as I had known them. Nothing more serious than a cold, or the occasional nasty flu that was going around. There was a time in Africa that my father suffered for a few days with a bout of malaria. I never saw a repeat of that episode however. We ate well. We ate lots of meat. My mother, being South American, served us meat for breakfast, lunch, and dinner. My mother was also a very Catholic woman. We ate fish every Friday. As long as I can remember, we had what is still considered a well-balanced diet. A protein, vegetable, and carbs. These ideas have come to change completely for me. I was not limited on the sugar either, but back then the sugar was just that, sugar. Today we have to deal with the ever-pervasive high fructose corn syrup. This was the lens through which I saw life. I never worried that both sets of grandparents met their makers at a rather young age and were all sick before their death. Each one had their own illness. Two of them had cancer. I was young then and did not think too far into the future. Fast forward a few years, and my father was showing signs of dementia. We could not put our finger on it but he was definitely slipping on an intellectual level. After a fifteen-year period he also started to hallucinate. He would see people that were threatening to him somehow. My father hated doctors and refused to see anyone. He had always been an athlete and had never stopped the habit of walking for hours every day. He was in good shape and "felt fine" physically. He had all his hair. He was tall and slim. He was a very well-dressed man. He refused to acknowledge he had any sort of problem. When we finally found a doctor—a neurologist friend of the family- to make a house call he diagnosed my father with Lewey Body Dementia. This is a very rare form of dementia. I loved my parents very much.

My mother was a beautiful woman that always had a sweet tooth. Just before my father had passed away in the hospital, my mother had complained of very strong headaches above her left eye. She had gone to several specialists and no one could figure out what was wrong with her. More than one of them had given her antibiotics saying she had a sinus infection more than likely. As it turned out, my mother had a brain tumor above her left eye that was causing a tremendous amount of pressure and almost closing her eye. The doctors decided on radiation therapy for the tumor. In the end, my mother was diagnosed with breast cancer, stage 4. She was 68, and otherwise a healthy woman. She had what we all considered at the time to be healthy eating habits. She was in good physical shape. She was happy traveling to visit her children every year. This is where I started my education.

I was facing the devastating reality that my parents were no longer with me and that they had left me a devastating genetic inheritance. My life had always been blessed and now I had to learn this difficult lesson. I had my two small children at the time and had already started to worry about what legacy I would leave them.

Water

A friend of mine had introduced me to the idea of Kangen water while my parents were still alive. I had also lived in Japan so I knew that the Japanese were always very advanced in their technology. Kangen water is ionized water produced through electrolysis. This was interesting. I started my path to discovery of so many things that caused me to change my life and that of my children.

The friend with the Kangen water had given me some recordings of a radio show about health. There were two men featured on this CD that were each experts in their field. One was a doctor that had come back from death's door and lived to educate us about it. The other was a biochemist that helped me to understand chemistry. The first doctor is an ophthalmologist (allopathic training) and ophthalmic plastic surgeon. After going through some harrowing experiences with illness, he discovered a way to heal the body through voltage. He was also the first person I had heard of that made the link between energy and the food we eat, acting as voltage. Reading his material, I came to discover that his principles were amazing. His explanation for any chronic pain in the body is low voltage. I learned to look at food. It surely stands to reason. The metaphor that has worked best for me to explain this idea is that of the automobile, my car does not run at all if I don't put gas in it. The difference is a human body can survive a limited time without fuel. We humans are resilient, until we aren't. That comparison is very simple and I think that's a good way for us to look at our bodies. If you put high quality gas in your car it will run better, smoother, and longer, if you take care of it. If you put high quality fuel in your body the same thing will happen. I studied with this doctor and became certified in his method of treating the body with his invention, the biomodulator. I achieved master status and always learned more with each class I took under him. He taught us that the basis behind Kangen water is alkalinity. This became a very important concept for me. The most important thing to remember about alkalinity is that cancer can't live in alkaline environments. Instead, cancer cells survive and even thrive in acidic environments.

I then attended an institute of health in West Palm Beach, Florida called Hippocrates Health Institute (HHI). I learned about food. The most important lessons HHI teaches is how to understand our relationship with food. Did you know that the average American diet is called SAD? It stands for Standard American Diet. Could that have been on purpose? This Western pattern diet is blamed for higher cases of obesity, heart disease, cancer, and more. As students of HHI, we learned about the nutrition available to us from food. We learned to think about what we were putting in our bodies. I remember the old saying "you are what you eat." I was amazed to know I was actually learning that this was completely true. During my time at HHI I also learned what it means to be vegan. I have been vegan for seven years now. That's right. I went from being a huge meat eater to vegan. I did it cold turkey as they say. I knew that if I wanted to benefit from this program of intense education, I needed to follow the program. I also wanted to understand what they would be teaching and what I would be teaching others eventually. Vegans do not eat anything with a face. That is the best way for me to explain to others what veganism is.

Over the years, veganism has been very misunderstood. As fad diets in the U.S. seem to be very popular, there was a time where lots of people were going vegan as they had heard things about it and wanted to join the movement (whatever it was). I hear this all the time from people. They invariably laugh at me after hearing that I'm vegan and say, "Yeah I tried that and I got sick." It isn't for me. When others say that to me, I know immediately that they did not educate themselves first on nutrition. They most likely made their decision based on what they thought might be cool or different. Realizing that the body needs nutrition and being able to supply your body with the energy it needs is vital. Through Hippocrates Health Institute, I became a certified health educator. I armed myself with as much education about food and nutrition for the body as I could. I also loved the term health educator, for I truly believe that is an important distinction. Give a man a fish, feed him for a day, teach him how to fish and you feed him for a lifetime. I live by this code and I believe we all have a right to education on our health. We all have the right to understand how our bodies work. I have never believed in leaving all the important decisions about health to the doctors. I had found my passion. Any extra weight I had on my body just seemed to fall off. I began looking for new and exciting things to eat as my meals had always been dominated by meat. I had incredible amounts of energy just like when I was younger.

I had always been an athlete, even after having my two children, I continued to learn new sports, finding my way to the martial arts. Before my education and career change, I was a karate teacher. I trained for nearly ten years in different martial arts styles. I even had my own classes. I had started my own small business teaching beginners karate to children and some self-defense classes to women. I always felt a calling to help others. During that time, I had been invited by a good friend to help with a mission in Africa. I grew up partially in Africa and I know that I wanted to be a part of this. My children were small and it was very difficult to be apart from them at the time. I served on the board of an NGO working in Liberia as the Gender Based Violence expert. The president of Liberia at the time was Ellen Johnson Sirleaf, a Harvard business graduate. We met with many government officials but what was most important to me was being able to teach self-defense classes while I was there, to the young women I could reach. All this to say that physical fitness was always a part of my life. I had learned that from my father. He had taught me how to be an athlete. I grew up playing every sport I could learn, and as a mother, in my thirties, I picked up martial arts. I already knew what exercise could do for health and the body. I probably reached the best shape of my life in my late thirties.

My work in nutrition and fitness led me to realize how much misinformation was out there for public consumption. One-minute coffee is being touted as good for you, the next it is bad for you. People I knew were constantly asking me questions about health and nutrition. I started to develop this interesting intuition about the health of others by just looking at them. It was almost like I could see what part of the body was not working properly. My work with other physicians and healers was enlightening me as to how the body would react in most situations. I had chosen to study physicians that were using knowledge of western medicine, and eastern medicine to create a more whole picture of the body. This information was starting to sink in and I was able to use it to help others. As I started to work with the ideas that this new ability brought me, I met my first client. He is now undoubtedly my best client. I qualify him this way as he has always had the ability to put into action any principle I teach him. In other words, he follows every instruction I have ever given him towards health. This student, we shall call him Adam, was not in the best of shape. Adam is a wealthy man that drank a lot, loved food, and was well into his fifties. He owned a yacht, a private jet, and had anything money could buy. He found me just as I was starting to work with clients to create a healthy lifestyle. He was interested in almost everything I had to teach him. This is where I learned that those at the top are usually there for a reason. I noticed that he had surrounded himself with experts in every field that was connected to him. He did not have the most basic idea of nutrition which I realize is not uncommon. Adam was amazing. He became a strict vegan. Everyone around him wondered what had happened to him and many of his friends made fun of him. He had adopted a new lifestyle and it was all about health. His sons were older and he worried about their health. He also started to give advice on health to those that would ask because I had taken the time to "educate" him on the why of everything I was recommending. Adam's first trip to the doctor he had been seeing for years was proof of my success as a health educator. He called me from his doctor's office and said that all his numbers were the best they had been in twenty years! His doctor was amazed. I had warned him not to say too much to his doctor about how he had changed his health so drastically. Adam's doctor merely said, "keep doing what you are doing." It has been a few years now since Adam has been my client, but we still keep in touch. He still calls me with questions, and every year he still calls me from his doctor's office thanking me for my help. I knew I was on to something from my success with Adam.

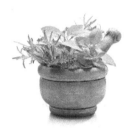

Chapter 3
Your Body Holds the Key

Understand Your Body and Heal Yourself

I t is important to have a critical mind when it comes to all the things we hear and see on TV for example. We must also realize that a doctor is also a human being. Some are good, and some are bad at what they do. There is a point in time that we understand how personal our own health is and that we are the only ones that really have any control over it. It will not be the doctor that cures you. It will be you. Your health and longevity is under your control. This is the big secret that no one wants you to know. We all like to think that there are institutions and organizations out there that exist to serve us, but the truth is that no one will take care of you as you can. Most large corporations, like the insurance industry and the pharmaceutical industries, are doing what they do for profit. If there were no profits, they would not be in business. Today, this profit has become enormous, and difficult to control. We no longer know who to trust. There are few regulations of these entities in our country. If we start to look closely, the individual with an illness becomes a cash cow. The more serious the illness, the more money this patient is worth. This makes me nervous. I saw this with the treatment and care of my parents.

Learning about health and longevity does not need to be a second career for everyone. Like Adam, it can be as easy as finding someone you trust with the knowledge that is relevant in today's world. There are many amazing products out there that are changing the face of healthcare. We are flooded with new technology and new science. Discovering new ways to treat the body with preventative medicine is a very exciting field. I have seen and studied so many new and non-invasive ways to recognize problems before they become disease, or illness that I am filled with hope for the future. All we have to do is reach out and learn.

Our Bodies Are Made Perfect

Establishing a pattern of health on a daily basis is key. Learn what is good for you and what is not. Our bodies were made perfect. We are designed to heal ourselves. The human body is a complex system that is incredibly efficient. We need to learn what the right things are in order to put them into our bodies. The reverse is also true. We need to know what is not right for our bodies. Although the latter is somewhat easier. When we find what's right for our bodies, we need to repeat it until we can see the difference working. Or rather feel the difference working. In this book you will learn the keys to health that fit into your life to bring you happiness and confidence knowing that you are living your best life.

How many times have you heard a doctor or even a dentist say, "oh it just means you are getting up there in age." There is nothing that gets me going more than someone in a position of authority saying this to another person. This is where critical thinking comes in. Never accept what others are saying unless you can ask questions and get answers that make sense. I will give you an example of this, when I was at the dentist just before turning fifty. I love my dentist, she is a beautiful person. I have confidence in her professional abilities as she helped me regain my smile where many dentists before her could not. She always listens and has the ability to think outside the box, mostly. I use the word mostly, this is why: As I was laying back in the chair in my dentist's office, I was waiting for her to come in and check my teeth after the hygienist did her thing. Now my dentist does know me and knows that I have an extra ordinary education in health. I had been noticing for some time that every time I ate, I had a tremendous amount of food stuck in my teeth afterwards. This had never been the case throughout my life, and the fact that it was happening now was strange to me. Nothing else had changed in my life for this experience to be so different all of a sudden. I do remember my American grandmother always sucking at her teeth whenever we went to visit her. I always thought it to be such an odious habit. Even as a little girl I knew the sound she made while sucking the food out of her teeth was not very nice to hear in public. I had vowed to never do that no matter what terrible thing might befall me in my old age. This was eye opening as I had recently started to make similar noises whenever I was done eating. I also used toothpicks all the time. So I asked my dentist, why I had this new problem for the past few years. My lovely dentist asked me if I had ever heard the expression, "long in the tooth." I almost fell backwards in surprise. I asked her if she meant to say that because I am getting older, my teeth were getting longer. She laughed and answered no, that it was actually the gums that start to recede after a certain age, in all of us. I asked her what actually caused gums to recede. There certainly isn't a magical age where that happens to all of us is there? It would necessarily depend on how well we take care of ourselves. Doesn't that stand to reason? I asked her if using bleaching agents such as the Crest white strips might cause some damage to the gums and cause them to start receding early. She replied yes, these bleaching agents were known to cause damage to the gums if they were applied too often or for longer than expressly instructed. This was something I had become addicted to a few years back when my children were still small. I loved to have white teeth as I finally had a smile I did not have to hide. We spoke about that for a few minutes and I realized that when people say something is an age thing, they are saying that because the possible explanations are too long and perhaps too involved to explain every time a patient would ask a question. Doctors simply do not have the time to share with us all the things we should know in order to properly take care of ourselves. The lesson here is always ask questions. You are paying for the service or time of that professional, you might want to insist on using it to your advantage. There are also a few more reasons why gums recede and they all have to do with nutrition. Our teeth are very important to our health. We must learn to pay extra attention to them and make sure we are taking them into account. I will discuss this further in Chapter 6.

The Immortal Cell

Science tells us that with proper care and nutrition, the cell is actually immortal. If the cell is immortal, then why do we age? There is a combination of things happening to cause our cells to degrade. A wise biochemist asked, "do you want your cells to reproduce out of recycled material, or new material?" I have never forgotten that explanation. Our cells reproduce. Each time a cell reproduces it divides into new cells. Each time it does that, it makes a copy of all the chromosomes which carry all of the instructions for life, sending a copy to the new cell. If we considered that every time we ate something, we might make different choices. We usually like to please our mouths only. We love the pleasure of the tastes, but we essentially pay later and keep on going. This is not critical thinking. We need to focus on what we want from life. I don't believe anyone that has been successful in business has given up the dream at any point in their career. There is a drive in all of those whom have risen to the top of their career fields and managed to stay there. Call upon this drive now to re-educate the body you have been given. We can literally remake ourselves. In fact, we do it all the time.

Have you ever heard that we regenerate ourselves every seven years? Well this is not exactly true. There is some truth to that statement and here is the skinny: Our skin takes about two to three weeks to renew itself. Our liver takes about 300-500 days to renew. Colon cells refresh after only four days. White blood cells take more than a year. Red blood cells are replaced very 120 days. A skeleton renews all bones in about ten years. There are some organs that stop growing after a certain time, like your brain. The cerebellum, or grey matter stops growing between two and three years of age. Our heart muscle stops growing at about ten-years-old as well. These two organs are the most important ones for us to live and have extra protection around them. As you can see, the health of our cells is vital to our health and our longevity. Again, we want to make sure our cells are renewing themselves with new material, and not recycled. There are some enlightened scientists and doctors that believe that all disease comes from malfunctioning cells. I have come to believe this as true. Everything is made up of cells. Cells each have their jobs to do. If one cell malfunctions and we are not healthy enough to discard that particular cell, then it will reproduce. If a malfunctioning cell is allowed to reproduce, it will continue until something goes wrong in our bodies. These changes will be happening in the body sometimes for a few years before it will be detectable to us. Therein lies the danger. We can literally reinforce our health and immune system to such a degree that we never risk even catching a cold. How do we work on this immune system of ours? How can we believe that we can reinforce our bodies to the point of never even being at risk of catching a cold? It is possible and I will explain how. With this information you will be able to fortify your amazing body to feel the way you deserve to feel all the time. When we know better, we do better, right!?

Food as Fuel

Our food is our fuel. If we don't fuel up, we don't run. Our human bodies will run for a time on empty, but not for long. One thing that we must remember is that our bodies are incredibly resilient. We can be sick for a long time before the body gives up. For now, we will focus on how to build a strong immune system no matter what. If food is our fuel, then it stands to reason that we must put a little effort into understanding what we should eat. When most of us eat, we do so for what delights our taste buds. Why not? We have taste for a reason, right? Yes, but the plot thickens. Our taste buds have been hijacked over the past few decades with the invention of many foods and additives that have been designed to fool our taste buds and have a specific effect on our brains. They also allow the processed foods to last much longer on our shelves, thereby improving the profit scale by untold amounts. Foods such as high fructose corn syrup and many of its derivatives that are under different names to fool us, are very bad for our health. A quick description of its evil powers are that it leads to insulin resistance which could lead to Type 2 diabetes. It can lead to obesity, heart disease, and wreaks havoc on our liver. Only liver cells can process fructose which causes the liver to start the over-production of fat. Fructose will also form tiny little holes in our intestinal lining which will most likely lead to "leaky gut." A leaky gut is when foreign food proteins and bacterial proteins slide through the intestinal walls directly into our blood streams where they don't belong. This leads to inflammation which leads to weight gain. Can you see where this is going? Weight gain that is uncontrolled, since you don't know what is going on most of the time, will lead to obesity and diabetes! All of this effectively increases your appetite as well. All of this happens because of a substance in our food that makes it taste better. Today we know that high fructose corn syrup is made with genetically modified corn (GMO). Whether you believe that GMOs are bad for you or not, you can already see the detrimental effect that high fructose corn syrup has on all of us. We must all learn to read labels. Try and eliminate all the foods you currently have in your home that contain this substance and consider the pervasive nature of it and how our ignorance has kept it in our lives.

High Voltage Food

Foods we do want in our bodies are what actually give us the voltage we need to have energy, think clearly, and basically function on every level. I will include liquid in a later chapter. For now we will learn about food. Did you know that each vegetable that we eat can give us voltage? A potato for example can produce up to five volts of energy. That is enough to light a small bulb. A lemon can produce .906 volts. Each vegetable and fruit has the capacity to produce energy. When we consume these things, we absorb the voltage. Our bodies use this to perform. Don't you want to perform your best? At least we all agree that we all want to feel our best, I hope. This is done through what we choose to eat. Consider this statement. Any pain we feel in our bodies is because we have low voltage in that area. Some of you may remember a book called *The Body Electric* by Robert O. Becker, an orthopedic surgeon that believed electromagnetism was the foundation of life. We all know that our heart's activity is coordinated by electrical impulses. Our entire bodies work on an intricate electrical system. Our cells are designed to run between a pH of 7.35 and 7.45. pH is a measurement of voltage. It really means potential hydrogen. Let me explain in more familiar terms. Our bodies are run by electricity. When we want our bodies to run smoothly, we need to put in the voltage we need to keep up our health. We get voltage from food. Voltage equals energy. The more voltage, the more energy we have in our bodies. So if cells can only make new cells out of the material you provide by eating, it's a certain voltage necessary to provide the energy needed to turn raw materials into new cells. Your body fights many minor battles every day in an effort to keep your body at 98.6° Fahrenheit. Any variation of this is a quick realization that something is wrong. Similarly, our pH balance is very important as well. We need a balance. The body is always striving for balance called homeostasis.

Knowing key facts about your body must be remembered at all times for you to heal yourself. You will be the only one held accountable. Remember the incredible human body was designed to heal itself. We only need to give it what it needs to heal and thrive. Always take care of your teeth as these are markers, among others, we need to pay attention to. They indicate where our attention should be. Taking care of our bodies on a cellular level is the primary reason we should learn how to eat. Optimally giving our cells raw materials, and not sub-standard materials to make new cells with. Our food is our fuel. The fuel we take in is the amount of voltage we have. The more voltage we have the more energy we have to heal as well as thrive.

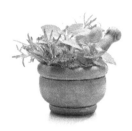

Chapter 4

You Are What You Eat

Maintain a Balance

E verything that we eat and drink has an effect on our alkaline/acid levels. You have learned that a perfect pH is 7.34, approximately. If it were possible to measure our pH levels every time we ate something, I think most of us would be surprised. Our pH levels fluctuate with what we eat and also the way we measure them also may have an influence, urine, blood, and saliva for example. Instead of measuring our pH levels constantly (which would not help us very much) we should look at the contents of what we decide to put into our mouths. What do we know about alkalinity and/or acidity? We know that human blood is maintained between pH 7.35 and 7.45 by acid-base homeostasis. Since this is true, it must be that there is a reason our bodies work on this balance. We also know that cancer does not live in alkalinity. Cancer needs an acidic environment to grow. We also know that animal proteins are very acidic. Meat, poultry, cheeses are acidic. Very sugary drinks like soda pops are very acidic. It's shocking but there is still controversy over these ideas, even though the medical community has ascertained that cancer thrives in an acid environment, and does not survive in alkaline environments. What would your choice be knowing these facts? There is a book published in 2006 that has an amazing explanation and study for nutrition, weight loss, and long-term health called *The China Study* written by T. Colin Campbell, PhD, and Thomas M. Campbell II, MD. This book is the most comprehensive study of nutrition ever conducted around the world. This book has been extremely controversial as it definitively points to our diets as the culprit to our nationwide (worldwide really) failing health. In it, Colin Campbell asserts that America's War on Cancer, started in the 1970s, has been a miserable failure. What business could last for over fifty years, with billions of dollars being funneled into it and still remain a failure? The business of cancer is the answer. We have not made any effective strides in the direction of cures, only of more questions. In fact, cancer has become more prevalent with time. The American Cancer Society says that men have a 47% chance of getting cancer and women have a 38% chance of getting cancer. Despite what we may have come to believe, cancer is not a natural event. Working on your diet and lifestyle is the best prevention of cancers and many illnesses in our society and world today. That is definitely the good news. The bad news is that you will have to decide what is more important to you, changing your diet, or battling an illness for the rest of your life. Prevention is key. Once we have been diagnosed with something, it becomes more difficult to get rid of what has taken hold of us. It is much easier to avoid getting something if we can understand the causes and how our bodies work.

I can't tell you how many times I have been asked by a waiter if I would like some protein with my salad. I always take the time to say that plants also have protein and that there is plenty of protein on my salad, thank you. Plant protein has a much more lasting effect on the body than animal protein. Compare it to the tortoise and the hare. Which one wins the race? The one that is slow but steady always wins. Plant protein has less of a punch, but lasts longer and is healthier to digest and absorb than meat. Plant protein is also alkaline. Meat is acidic and takes much longer to digest than plants. Meat can also make you feel very tired and sluggish after eating. There is much proof by way of the athletes today that are choosing a vegan diet over meat to fuel their athleticism and competition. The Iron Man Triathlon, considered the most difficult one-day endurance event in the world, has a few vegans to boast. The key is health and endurance again. I am a true believer as I have been both a huge meat eater and now a vegan.

Our bodies need to have a balanced pH level at all times. It is definitely advantageous to have a slightly more alkaline state than acidic state. Meat and cheeses are acidic. More alkaline foods will help the body avoid illness. When I made the choice to be vegan and studying at HHI, I noticed a few changes. One was I had no idea what to eat most of the time. While I was there, we had the advantage of the cafeteria that had the best tasting food and they served strictly raw vegan. I had never been a lover of salads, or vegetables for that matter. I was always surprised at the tastes they could achieve with just plants. It was a whole new world for me. I noticed that my body was changing as well. I was in my late thirties and in good shape, but I had been gathering a few pounds that were not there before and very difficult to get rid of. In fact, impossible. When I got to Hippocrates and became vegan, the extra weight just seemed to slip off. I have always been relatively thin, but I actually weighed the same as in high school without even trying. I also felt some strange thickness in my joints as I continued my vegan journey with my class. I asked a few other classmates if they felt the same as it was not a good feeling for me. It made me feel weak and I was still hitting the gym lifting weights when I was not in class. Our resident personal trainer for cruise ships, a twenty-six-year-old Australian that was in class with us, told me to keep going, that the feeling would subside. He explained that he too had felt the same way (he was in better shape than me) a few weeks into the new diet. He explained that it was the excess animal proteins, that felt like they were clogging my joints, leaving my body. It was a slow, sticky feeling and did not last. By the three-week period of my nine weeks stay at

HHI, I was feeling amazing. I had newfound energy. I felt a mental clarity that was a little scary to tell you the truth. I just felt so good and never really missed meat at all.

Vitamins and Supplements

Whenever we make a decision to change something in our diet, we must do so responsibly. We need to make sure that we are giving the body all the things it needs to be strong and healthy. From animal proteins we do get a few things we need easier and faster than other foods. In my opinion, the price of getting it through meat is too high a price. I choose to educate myself and find alternatives for these nutrients that do not have any negative effects at all. In doing so, I have found that my diet does not lack anything. I choose to educate myself instead of just cutting something completely out of my diet. This is an important point. I have had friends tell me that they were vegan for a while but they stopped because they got sick. Well this is not an educated way to do something. If you are avoiding something in your diet in order to balance out your body, then you must replace things you need with another source. An example of this is B vitamins. We get B vitamins from proteins like fish, poultry, meat, eggs, and dairy products. Leafy green vegetables, beans, and peas also have B vitamins. There are also great B vitamin supplements we can take to keep our balance. Education is key! You have learned that food is what supplies our voltage. Plants give us voltage to feed our cells, and meat takes voltage in order to be digested properly. Yes, when we eat meat, it takes more energy for our bodies to digest it. It takes 20-30% of the total calories in a piece of meat to digest it. Fruits and vegetables actually donate energy to the body. We are able to use these calories as energy. The time food takes to travel through the gastrointestinal tract is also of importance as we have seen lots of problems with the gastrointestinal tract in this country. The more fiber in our food, the less time it takes to travel through our bodies. Only plants have fiber. The meat eaters take up to 24 hours longer for their food to travel through their colons. From these facts we must make our decisions to either live a long and healthy life, or subject ourselves to the pleasures of the mouth and suffer the consequences, whatever they may be. We all have free will. We all have the ability to reason. Let's use it.

The subject of supplements is one that is best left to the experts, unless you are a researcher. What makes the most sense to me is to eat as much nutrition as we can, so we really don't need to spend all day taking pills. I used to take lots of supplements every day. I spent a fortune on them as well. No one can take lots of pills every day and not get sick of it eventually. I learned that the companies that produce vitamins and supplements mostly put fillers in them with very little of the actual vitamin. Again, this equals more profits for the makers. All supplements are not made equal.

It is important to know which company out there is invested in improving our health and which company is just looking to turn as much profit as they can. What I have learned is that eating whole foods and not taking as much supplements is the best way to go. When we eat foods, we not only get the vitamins, we get so much more. We get all the nutrients available in that particular food. When we take a pill, we get very little of that vitamin and also some of the things they put in as fillers. This is an added danger. Not what we want.

Raw Foods

Eating raw foods is especially important. When we don't cook food, we preserve the natural enzymes (and voltage) in the food. We need and benefit from these enzymes. When we cook our veggies, we tend to cook out most of the nutrients, like the enzymes. Enzymes are defined as a substance produced by a living organism that acts as a catalyst to bring about a specific biochemical reaction. Another description that helps us understand the importance of enzymes can be that a cell is really just some chemical reactions that are made possible by enzymes.

Our cells are constantly working for us. We are a collection of cells, as is everything. If our cells need enzymes to perform, then shouldn't we be replenishing them as often as we can? It is not just salads that we need to eat. It is also fruit, nuts, anything that tastes good without cooking it. All raw foods contain enzymes. We must make an effort to incorporate raw foods into our diets every day. These enzymes help us to digest our food in order to distribute the nutrients to the rest of our bodies. There are also enzymes found in foods such as sauerkraut, which is considered a fermented food. Fermented raw foods are considered a probiotic.

Probiotics are important for us to maintain a balance of bacterial flora in our gut. Without this, we may suffer if we have ever taken an antibiotic for an infection or a virus. Antibiotics kill every bacteria, even the good ones. There was a time when a doctor used to prescribe probiotics every time an antibiotic was prescribed. This practice is no longer advised unfortunately. If we don't maintain a balance of bacteria in our guts, we may be overrun by some bad bacteria. There are a few places bacteria can hide in our bodies undetected. We want to avoid this. By eating a probiotic every day we can learn to maintain a healthy relationship with bacteria in our bodies and maybe even eliminate bloating if we manage to find our intestinal balance! Wouldn't that be nice! I know a man that is about eighty-something years old, and carries a bottle of enzymes with him wherever he goes. He would pull out a bottle of capsules, pop a few into his mouth and chew them raw. "Like candy" is what he would say. When we decide to eat cooked food, we can also put some enzymes on our cooked food to help us digest properly avoiding any issues with bloating for example, and consequently any problems in the future. Enzymes can be bought in capsule form making it easy to sprinkle on food we are eating.

A Balanced Diet

While learning about food and nutrition, I found out that the combination of food was just as important as deciding on what was the best diet for our health. Our stomachs have a process to digest each and every thing we eat. When we combine the wrong things together, we cause problems. I always thought that having a protein (meat, nuts, and seeds), a vegetable, and a carb would be a balanced meal. After all, that is what we were taught growing up isn't it? I was wrong. Learning how to combine food helps us reduce the taxation of our digestive processes. The proper food combinations are to never mix certain foods such as meat and potatoes. Yes, it's true. This could be a huge factor in the collective weight gain of Americans, among other things. We must learn to combine proteins with the right carbs. For example when eating meat or animal protein, we should combine with a vegetable. The best carb-rich foods are unprocessed foods from plant sources. This includes whole grain side dishes, like couscous, brown rice, barley, oats, quinoa, etc. An easy way to remember the proper food combining is this: proteins with veggies or carbs with veggies. Remembering this can relieve many issues for our digestive experience.

What Is Indigestion?

The next important factor when thinking about the health of the gut is hydrochloric acid. Generally speaking, we are able to digest our food in our gut with the help of hydrochloric acid (HCL). In order to produce HCL we need iodine, zinc, and B1 vitamins. When we do not have enough of these ingredients, and we have suffered abuse to the digestive tract from lack of knowledge, we might be feeling what has become known as reflux. Acid reflux is simply the formation of gas bubbles from not having enough stomach acid. Yes, you read that correctly. It is easy to buy HCL and aid our bodies in the formation of HCL in order to properly digest our food and avoid further problems. When we take antacids, we are effectively cutting off our own ability to make HCL even further, causing more problems. Stomach acid kills what we will call "bugs" in our food. There are many types of bacteria that are potentially harmful to the body that we come into contact with every day. If we don't have enough HCL we become defenseless to the bugs in our food as it goes down the hatch. Our bodies can't absorb zinc without stomach acid. If we don't have zinc, we can't make dopamine and serotonin. If we can't produce these things in our bodies, we may suffer from depression among other things. This is an example of how our bodies are amazingly sensitive and need to constantly strive for balance. There are certain things that will block the absorption of zinc, and caffeine is one of them. When drinking coffee or black tea, we should be waiting before we eat any nutrition.

There is also a hidden danger in the majority of painkillers we find on the market, such as aspirin. We seem to be ignorant of the dangers associated with these over the counter medications and suffer the consequences without even knowing why. Even one small aspirin is known to create a tiny hole in your stomach lining which will bleed. Over time you can imagine the damage. The good news, beyond the fact that we are amazingly resilient beings, is that we can help cure this problem and many others for that matter, with the use of Vitamin C. I, and many of the physicians I have studied with, love Vitamin C. It is a very potent anti-oxidant that we could all use in our lives, and it will eventually heal the lining of your stomach among many other things.

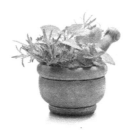

Chapter 5

The Mystery of Water

The Benefits of Water

Of all the things I learned, the most interesting subject is Water. None of us really fully understand water. If anything is touted as the elixir of life, I believe it to be water. Our bodies are made of about 60% water. Amazing! All that liquid in your body. Water is another substance that is absolutely necessary for us to live. There is a lot of controversy about water. In the United States we have come up with some pretty amazing products relating to water. If we delve further, it is important to understand the idea of alkaline water as essentially water with an added charge. In other words, electrons have been added. There are a few ways to do this, but first let's start with why. The best explanation is the origin. What I discovered was that the Russians were the first to work on the idea of adding electrons to water. I was told a version of this to be that the Russians were experimenting with the idea of alkaline water to help their astronauts heal as they returned from their mission to outer space. They were using a process of electrolysis to separate the molecules of water, which later became part of the process of forming alkaline water. It is on record that the Russian scientists were working with the Japanese to better perfect the process of electrolysis and make alkaline water. The Japanese quickly saw the benefits of this water. Since then there have been many theories about alkaline water and its many health benefits.

I made a reference earlier in Chapter 2 about the process of electrolysis as not being the best way to make alkaline water. There are those of us that have heart conditions they must live with and be aware of. One of them is atrial fibrillation, or afib. It is an irregular, rapid heart rate that can cause symptoms like shortness of breath, palpitations, and fatigue to name a few. It is not always dangerous but it certainly can be. Since we know that it is electricity that makes our hearts beat, drinking alkaline water made by the use of electrolysis would be harmful over time for someone with afib. One of the theories that started the research came from a famous tribe called the Hunza. They are one of the longest living people on Earth today. One of the theories about their famed longevity is that their water source was that of natural alkaline water from the mountains. Water as pure as it should always be for us. Mineralized, alkaline, and vital, from the Himalayas. Their diet, of course, is also free of any preservatives, given their distance from most of civilization. Today there are many companies that sell what is called Kangen water made by machines using the process of electrolysis. There are other companies I have found that have really nailed the way to produce alkaline water in its purest form. It is available to all of us that understand what this is worth to our lives, families, and our health. The most important thing to understand is that we all need clean drinking water. Today, the world is suffering from a lack of clean water. There are places that still do not have access to clean water. Before we go and count ourselves as the lucky ones, let's look at our water. In the United States going back to around 1962, it was mandated to add fluoride in the water. There is still great controversy over this today. I know that in the state of Florida, it is the county that decides whether to add fluoride or not. Originally it was determined that adding fluoride was necessary for the prevention of tooth decay. Today we know a little more about fluoride and many are against it being added to our water supply. Fluoride is considered a toxic substance as it can kill if ingested in certain quantities. That's why the toothpaste containers are all labeled "keep out of reach of children." There is a danger that children might eat toothpaste because of its good taste. Ingesting fluoride can kill you. Today we have so many fluoridated products that some argue we really don't need it in our water anymore. This seems obvious so why is it not stopped? The truth is somewhere out there. I am not one to wait for any government to declare what is good or bad for me. By the time these decisions are made, we have already forgotten about the problem. I have seen what can happen when too much fluoride is ingested and it is not pretty.

The Dangers in Our Water Supply

My family used to live in Kenya. When I first got to Nairobi, I noticed all the African kids at my school had brown teeth with pieces missing. I was so shocked I asked someone why this was so. A man that worked with my father blithely answered, the Kenyan government had put too much fluoride in the water and this was the result. We, as foreigners, were warned never to drink tap water. It is also known that fluoride can cause the calcification of our pineal gland. Our pineal gland is what regulates our circadian rhythm helping us with our sleep habits. It also regulates reproductive hormones. The pineal gland is known as our third eye. This is where many people believe our intuition exists. Expanding consciousness and keeping our bodies vibrant and healthy sound pretty important and I would suggest keeping the pineal gland fluoride free.

Besides fluoride, there are still more hidden dangers in our public water supply. Prescription drugs are also a problem. My children came back from a field trip to the water treatment plant of our area, and told me to never throw any pills or prescriptions in the toilet. I laughed at first, then got the full story. They had been told upon leaving the educational tour that the biggest contamination and the hardest thing to remove from the water supply was drugs. The workers at the water plant were trying to reach the parents. Never throw drugs down the toilet as they will end up in your own water supply. Today, even reverse osmosis water filtration systems can't boast a completely pure water supply because of the difficulty in removing drugs from the water. The companies out there that produce pure water are only allowed to claim 99.9% pure due to this problem. Still, 99.9% is great for me. There are companies that produce clean, structured, alkaline, and remineralized water. This is undoubtedly the best as it is the closest to nature.

Let's look at the term structured. Why would water be structured? Water seeks structure. A molecule of water in the public water supply is large. It has many things attached to it. Besides fluoride and drugs, there is also the addition of chlorine for disinfecting purposes, etc. Each of these that are added to the water supply attach themselves to the molecule of water and goes with the flow. (By now you might have appreciated my layman terms for the science I am attempting to explain.) I believe when we know the reasons for things, we are able to grasp them better and they become our own. A simple molecule of water going into the water supply, becomes larger as these other existing materials attach themselves to the water on a cellular level. The molecule of water becomes large. Think of a magnet with all kinds of metallic objects sticking to it on all sides. A pure water molecule is not normally carrying such "baggage" if you will. A pure water molecule is much smaller and has the potential to hydrate your whole body. If the molecule is larger, it will not be able to pass everywhere it should within our bodies. We all have what is called a blood brain barrier. It is designed to keep one of our most important organs, the brain, safe from attacks going on within the body. A molecule that is too large, becoming unrecognized or foreign, is kept from passing this barrier. If we are only drinking water from the tap, with no attempt to filter it, we are certainly not receiving enough hydration for the brain. Remember how much of our body is water! We need to be hydrated. It is vital for our health and longevity.

There is an illness making itself known around the world more and more, it's called brain degenerative disease. One such killer is Alzheimer's. There are many more that affect the brain but this seems to be more common around the world. It is attacking younger and younger victims. The best attempt at avoiding any problems that could possibly come from not enough hydration is to use a reverse osmosis filtration system as it removes the most impurities. Only using r.o. is not the solution however. Reverse osmosis produces unstructured water. The process used to detach and eliminate the extra additives to water leaves the water molecules unstructured. Again, water seeks structure. If water is left unstructured it will find minerals to bond with in your body. As they continue to bond, they will eventually flush out the minerals. This is not advisable. The same is true for distilled water. Distilled water is pure and therefore unstructured. It will leech out minerals wherever they can be found. We want to hold on to our minerals and continue to add more, not have them flushed out of our bodies with the water we are drinking. It is not simple. Chemistry was never my favorite subject, but now it is infinitesimally more interesting. Reverse osmosis is only helpful if we find a way to structure the molecule of water after. Adding an extra ionic charge to make it alkaline, and remineralizing it naturally sounds like the perfect water doesn't it? There are companies that produce exactly that. This perfect water will also hydrate the brain. The molecular structure is small enough to pass through the blood brain barrier. Now we need to focus on the dangers that exist in the choice of materials used to transport and distribute water around the world.

Killer Plastic

There have been many studies done on the plastic containers used to house water for sale and distribution. It seems the world has realized that tap water is not as beneficial or clean. Now, the problems we face are in the water bottles. When plastics are exposed to heat and/or cold the structure of the plastic changes. For the purposes of education I will keep it simple. As water bottles sit waiting for distribution, in their plastic containers, they are exposed to many temperature changes. This might be dependent upon where they are stored, the temperature of where they are stored, and also the transportation system that will distribute them. If they are exposed to heat or freezing temperatures, the plastic from the bottle will leech out into the water. No matter how pure our water may be once it is poured into a plastic container it will change with time if exposed to climate changes. These changes are not good ones. Once the chemicals in plastic have leeched into the water, they will in turn affect our own cells as we drink this water. Our cells effectively could become plasticized. Our cells have an outer membrane that controls the movement of substances going in and out. It is permeable to ions and to organic molecules. It also regulates how much of any substance goes in. It also helps to support the cell and help maintain its shape. When we expose our bodies to the plastics and/or polymer composites used in construction, we are affecting our cells. Studies such as NHANES (the National Health and Nutrition Examination), designed to assess the health and nutritional status of adults and children in the U.S., have shown the existence of plastics among other chemicals in the general population. We are essentially plastifying our cell walls into being too hard, or too soft. Whatever the case may be, either is undesirable and may cause toxicity to the point of disease. The plastic in polymers act like estrogen in our bodies causing hormonal imbalances and also blocking zinc. Some of the plastics to watch out for are: bisphenol A, phthalates, styrene, acrylamide, triclosan, and brominated flame retardants. Even when these substances are labeled bad and there is public outcry, new ones are produced to put in their place and the event starts all over again. Eventually we find out again that they too are bad for our health. In 2008, a report issued by the U.S. National Toxicology Program (NTP) expressed concern for effects on the brain, behavior, and prostate gland in fetuses, infants, and children at what was the current human exposure to bisphenol A. There was also a minimal concern for effects on mammary glands in female fetuses, infants, and children at the current rate of exposure for the same bisphenol A. Later it was also found to be guilty of potentially causing obesity. The only reason these substances are being invented and used is to make things last longer, therefore bigger profits for the manufacturer. Our health is not a main concern for manufacturers of processed food. Everywhere I go I make sure I have glass bottles of drinking water. I do not compromise in this, for myself nor for my children. It is important to determine which things we decide are available to us and our particular genetics, and which things are not. I have breast cancer in my direct lineage, therefore I choose to never take a chance at all with my health by drinking from a plastic bottle.

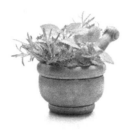

Chapter 6

Markers of Good ... or Bad Health

"Grandma, why are your teeth so long?"

By now hopefully you have figured out my pattern of linking how the body works and what your influence is as the person in charge of it. I have always been motivated by understanding. The more I understand, the more I can picture the best possible outcome and program myself for it.

We all carry so much information that has been programmed in us almost without exception. It can be difficult sometimes to distinguish between our own opinions or what we are pushed to believe by the media, society, culture, and even language. When I started to seriously study health, I traveled to seminars, master classes, courses, and conventions. The more I learned, the better I felt. I had changed my lifestyle and I really could feel the difference. I am a positive person by nature, but I knew over time I had slowly started to settle in small ways, compromising my body and health. Those small compromises can become large problems down the road. Once I understood more about food, my own body, and my genetics, it became easier to look for ways to feel better and better.

There are a few markers in the body that have been shown to be linked to our ability to heal. One such marker is our teeth. Each one of our teeth sits on a meridian line, or energy line running along our bodies. If there is problem, or interruption of the energy flow through your body, you will begin to show signs. Dental health is incredibly important. In 1923, Dr. Weston Price wrote 1,174 pages, two volumes, on research that took about twenty-five years to complete. His research was on a very high percentage of chronic degenerative diseases that could potentially originate from root filled teeth. In 1915, the American Dental Association appointed Dr. Price as their first Research Director. His advisory board represented fields of bacteriology, pathology, rheumatology, surgery, chemistry, and cardiology. Dr. Price was proving his theory on focal infections. The focal infection theory asserts that germs from a central focal infection, like teeth, roots, gums, even tonsils, could metastasize to hearts, eyes, kidneys, lungs, and other organs. Even glands and tissues could be affected. This was new and radical information at the time, but now has been proved and demonstrated over the years.

About seventy years ago the American Dental Association buried this information, affecting dentistry ever since.

Today most people, doctors, and patients, believe that infections are less dangerous since we now have antibiotics. Here is the problem with that line of thinking. A root filled tooth no longer has a direct blood supply. A root canal is essentially the absence of a root. The tooth is removed with its root, then replaced with a substitute. This can be done in different ways. What is important to understand is when a root is removed, the tooth itself is considered a dead tooth. It is no longer connected to a blood supply and stands on its own as dead tissue. A tooth structure includes microscopic tubules running through the dentin, which supply fluid (nourishment) to the inside of the tooth. If a tubule of a front single root tooth were stretched out straight, it would run about three miles. If we were to be prescribed antibiotics for a root canal, the antibiotics would not affect the rootless tooth as it is no longer connected to the body. There is no way for any fluid, let alone the antibiotics to get to the tooth. The bacteria present however, will literally be able to migrate through the blood stream, the preferred mode of transport, to any other unsuspecting location in the body. To explain this in simple terms for those of us that are not dentists: when a root canal is performed, there is usually something wrong with the tooth. If this is so, it will more than likely have bacteria present. This bacteria could easily, and usually, be in the area of the affected tooth, like the surrounding tissues and bone. Just removing the tooth will not necessarily eliminate the bacteria. The dead tooth, itself considered dead tissue, still has bacteria in it. If this same tooth is put back into the mouth, we can expect it to become infected. It is not a question of if, but when. Any dead tissue should always be removed from the body. Just pulling a tooth is not enough. There is a special technique that can be performed that makes sure to remove all the affected area and some effective ways to encourage infection free healing. Even teeth that show no indication whatsoever of any problems or infections can still contain bacteria that will not show up in any detectable way and cause havoc in the body. In many patients that were treated by Dr. Price, their illnesses would vanish as soon as the offending tooth was simply removed completely. Patients with crippling arthritis living in wheelchairs, with no visible problems in their root canals, were walking a few days after the removal of the tooth. Each tooth sits on one end of a circuit that flows through your body in a certain path. This path can be traced to treat and heal what the problem has become once the tooth has been taken care of. These circuits have different names, but they mostly follow the ancient lines of acupuncture that have been mapped out to show the energy flow through the body and organs.

This knowledge only helps us to keep ourselves in good health when it comes to knowing what to look for. We are called to either look for the right doctor we can see eye to eye with, or to seek out an ally that has this information and can help us figure out where to start looking for the solution. Knowledge of meridian lines is also vital to helping us understand how to heal ourselves. We need to become aware of our energy flow in order to better understand how to keep the flow steady and balanced. The East Asian arts of understanding this flow are extremely intricate as they have been studying this art for centuries. One of them is acupuncture. Most of us have an idea of what acupuncture is but maybe the understanding of why and how it works is not completely clear to us yet. We westerners are becoming more familiar and respectful of the knowledge held by Eastern Asia. The body has different wiring systems. One of them is the analog perineural nervous system and the other is known as the acupuncture system. They are both made of fibrous tissue. The first controls the conscious mind and the autonomous nervous system. These wiring systems are made of fibrous tissue. We call this our fascia. It is a network or web of tissue that extends from head to toe in all directions of your body covering everything. It is uninterrupted. When we have good energy flow through these networks, or systems, we are in good shape. When there is a problem, maybe something just starting to take hold, we feel a shift in energy of the body. If we do not have the vital energy we need to take care of the problem, we need to know how to increase this energy flow to hit the right spots for the right amount of time. For acupuncture, there is a belief that if something stops, or interrupts the flow of energy through your body it will cause a backup or imbalance. Small needles placed appropriately are believed to redirect the flow of your energy to heal. There are many words known for this life force, or energy. Chi is the Chinese word for energy force. This is a vital energy we must hold on to and work with. This is also believed by many different cultures as a way to heal. Mapping out these flows of energy, or meridian lines, we investigate how we can heal everything. When we see a stop or block in the flow, we can trace these back to an organ and find a way to add voltage and treat this affected area once the energy flow has been corrected. Again, diet plays an important part in delivering the raw materials needed for our cells to function the way they are meant to. There are rules that mother nature has set which all things natural follow. To understand these rules is to understand a part of life that we all have to work with. These meridian lines can all be traced throughout our bodies. Another way to help the flow of energy, or increase the flow of energy, is to add electrons to the body. Nutrition equaling voltage is electron energy. Alkaline or ionized water is also an electron donor. When we add this voltage to our problem, correct the energy flow, we are well on our way to healing most things we can think of.

Skin Deep

The next marker we can learn about is our skin. Our skin is the most overlooked organ in the body and it is huge. It covers all of us, and is incredibly resilient. It is an excellent indicator of what could be wrong. We often ignore our skin, expecting it to return to normal as always. These signs are indicators the we must always listen to. From the lines on our face from the pillow at night to the red rash we get from certain allergies. Each one is unique to its body and indicates how we are doing or handling things internally. When we feed ourselves well, our skin glows. When we neglect our bodies and forego real nutrition, our skin shows it. One of the most important things we need for our skin and our gut (immune system) is omega fatty acids. They are polyunsaturated fats that are essential. The brain, the nervous system, the liver, and every cell membrane are made of fats. We need good fats to keep making our cells strong and healthy. They are highly recommended by the physicians interested in helping us heal. Omega fatty acids come in three different types, 3's, 6's, and 9's. Each one is important and also the combination, as you have already learned, is very important. I recommend getting omega fatty acids from plant sources. You simply can't go wrong there. There are many recommendations on television offering omega supplements from fish sources. The omega that are derived from fish are mostly derived from fish liver, which brings me to the next marker to look for, the liver. When the liver is affected, our skin will usually show signs. Our liver's main job is to filter blood coming from the digestive tract before it goes to the rest of our bodies. Our liver plays a central role in our bodies. It breaks down fats and uses them to produce energy. It also breaks down old and damaged blood cells. Essentially the liver's job is to clean up. In reference to the omega source, would you want to eat omega fatty acids that have come from the liver of a fish that is contaminated? We now know that our world's fish supply is also contaminated. In studies reported by an article in the journal *Annals of Internal Medicine* from December of '04, the overconsumption of certain fish is harmful and can cause neurological deficits. Among the problems listed are cancer, autoimmune diseases, endocrine disorders, and even heart disease. The pollutants affecting this contamination are industrial, as well as consumer, including toxins like mercury, and polychlorinated biphenyls (PGBs). Extremely toxic substances. When we eat the fish, we also consume the same toxins existing in the fish. These toxins may have much the same effect on our bodies as they have on the fish.

A human liver has great tasks to perform and is often taxed. I have read countless books and theories of healers that say all pain or problems in the body can be moderated if not healed completely by cleansing the liver. This is an interesting idea as our livers are mainly responsible for cleaning or purifying our bodies. It would make sense if our liver is not able to clean up as intended, we might be suffering some effects of this inefficiency. If our liver is not successful at what it is meant to do, there must be a reason. Remember the liver replaces itself every 300-500 days. If we were suffering some kind of blockage where our liver was not working properly, the ability to help the liver cleanse itself would be a solution that has a great chance of improving our entire situation. The difficulty would be finding the right cleanse. There is so much information out there that it is vital to know what information you can trust. A very important point to know about the liver that will help us tremendously to understand our bodies better is how it cleans itself, how it actually gets ready to do its most important task of purifying the body. Remember where you read that the good kinds of cholesterol were good for the body? The liver actually makes cholesterol in order to clean itself. Yes, it makes cholesterol in reaction to overuse, or toxicity if you will. If your doctor has found your cholesterol level too high, he would interpret a few things from this. One would be that your diet is too high in saturated fats and your body is unable to process this successfully (as well it shouldn't), and that your liver is being taxed in its effort to clean itself to continue serving you. In a doctor's office, you would be prescribed something to lower your cholesterol level, which directly interrupts the process of your liver doing its job. In turn, hopefully you understand if you choose to continue eating bad fats, you will potentially incur chronic disease until you can figure out how to understand correctly what goes on inside that magnificent body of yours. This is, in fact, a clear explanation as to how chronic problems may arise. When people say it's because we are getting old, it makes me want to sit down with them and explain all the things I know about the body. The problem is not age. The problem is how we have chosen to live for the years we have been alive. As some of you read this, there might be the instinct to feel overwhelmed and regretful of the choices we have made in the past. There is no reason to fear, as you are a resilient creature. To love your body with knowledge and clarity is always the best way to recover your vitality and reverse any aging process that might be underway at any point in our lives. No point in regret, as to know better is to do better, right?!

Thyroid

The next marker to look for in our attempt to trace any interruptions to our life force is the thyroid. The markers I have mentioned are ones that are most common in our population. These are most likely where all of our illnesses mostly stem from. It is impossible to make a blanket statement about health as it is so individual to our environment and our individual diets, but overall, these markers are the best places to start cleaning up and getting to the foundations of our health. The thyroid is part of our endocrine system. The major endocrine glands are the thyroid and the adrenal glands. These glands work together to keep us going. The thyroid is found on both sides of the neck below the Adam's apple. It secretes thyroid hormones that influence our metabolic rate and protein synthesis. It has an effect on many things in our bodies including development. The most common problem that arises is an iodine deficiency.

There is a theory among the holistic doctors I have studied with that traces, in part, our epidemic of thyroid problems in the U.S. back to the dentist again. At least twice a year for most of us, our dentist subjects us to x-rays aimed at the mouth and consequently to the throat. Radiation in any dose that we expose ourselves to consistently is not good. We get it from the sun, from traveling on planes at high altitudes, from airport security, etc. There is only so much that our bodies can handle well. The x-rays at the dentist twice a year aimed at our naked throats, are believed by some to be overkill. They were invented for a reason and I have never heard a physician say they were unnecessary. However, for us to be the purveyor of what we think we need and how much, is a call for us all to make individually. We can do that by asking questions. I frequently ask my dentist if it is necessary this visit, and often ask her to forego the x-rays if both she and I agree that there is nothing really out of the ordinary at the time of my visit. I go at least two to three times a year and make sure that I let her know if there is any change she should be aware of.

There are different signs to look for in how to spot a thyroid that is unhealthy. The most important way besides a blood test, which is not always accurate, is to test your basal temperature. Basal temperature is what you measure when the body is at rest. We all know that a normal temperature in a balanced body is 98.6 or close. (If you are a red head you may have a slightly higher temperature). A pretty accurate way to test your basal temp is to keep a thermometer next to your bed. As soon as you wake up, test your temperature and write it down. Do this four or five days in a row and you have an average basal temperature. If it varies from the 98.6, either higher or lower, you might be experiencing thyroid fluctuations. There are a few other signs I have learned from the experience of the physicians I studied and they are quick to spot. If someone suffers from hyperthyroidism, a symptom can be large, bulgy round eyes. Sudden or extreme, often uncontrollable weight loss and weight gain are also signs. Some of these signs and more become what some holistic doctors use to check off all the boxes when looking at how to start eliminating possibilities and quickly find where the body is ailing. If you feel that there is an imbalance after looking at markers and finding some differences, then you have to find out how to correct the problem. Supplementing your diet with iodine is easy to do. Iodine is a naturally occurring chemical. In small doses it can help support your thyroid. In large doses it can be poisonous. There is small amounts of iodine in food as well, but not enough to harm the body.

Today the trace iodine in foods has mostly been processed out, which might help explain the number of increased thyroid problems the U.S. faces.

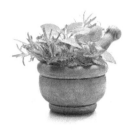

Chapter 7
We Are All Toxic

Toxins in Our Environment

T he world is and will always be a beautiful place. As we experience life and grow, we learn to choose which way we want to see things. Are you a glass half full kind of person, or the opposite? Either way, there is always beauty to behold. We just have to keep an eye out for it. Our environment is not always what we choose for ourselves no matter how successful we become. Adaptability and grace are needed to move through life and learn our lessons. This is true for the individual as well as the society we live in, no matter where on Earth you live. The state of our environment can be directly traced to the speed of our technological advancement, and our society's need for immediate results or gratification. We have indulged so much that now it is seen as a way of life, or a way to be. Today we are suffering the consequences. In my studies, I found books that described the toxicity in our lives and what it was doing to our environment and consequently to our bodies

There are statistics that show even a newborn baby is born with some toxicity. It stands to reason since a fetus receives the nourishment it needs to grow and develop through the mother. The fetus has already been exposed, albeit in a secondhand way, to the exterior world's problems. Anything the mother eats or drinks, the child is exposed to. Once this baby is born, he or she is promptly submitted to a combination of vaccinations deemed appropriate by our government and pediatricians.

One of the keys to our survival is to be aware of our surroundings and acknowledge how many of these contaminants can be avoided, and which ones can be mitigated. In a book by John Robbins called Diet for a New America, he says, "We produce pesticides today at a rate more than 13,000 times faster than we did 35 years ago." These numbers do not seem far-fetched when we consider the rate of plastic products being produced, the pharmaceuticals, hormones, and other additives in our food, etc. We have become used to this knowledge but what is this combination of toxins doing to us? We have more cases of autism than ever before. We see more and more cancer. Brain degenerative diseases are becoming more common. Autoimmune diseases are also on the rise. Our bodies can't always recognize what we are putting in to our bodies if it has nothing from nature in it. If our cells can't recognize it, they can't use it. They are then not capable of regenerating new cells. We need to find a way to lessen our toxic burden.

Avoiding things like high fructose corn syrup, genetically modified foods, saturated fats, reducing or eliminating animal protein, and basically all processed food, is important and should be something we work at getting perfect at some point in our lives. But what do we do if we find ourselves fifty and over, picking our heads up for the first time to finally start enjoying the moment, the world around us, and the hard work we have done to create a piece of heaven for ourselves and our generations to come?

Whether or not you think you're toxic is no longer the question. The question has become how toxic! We look for the markers and work on understanding what is happening in the body to try and correct it. We want to eventually feel like we are starting with a clean slate, I have witnessed amazing transformations in people dedicated to their new healthy lifestyle. Your biological age should show your health not your numerical age.

Anything we do toward incorporating healthful habits is a step towards detoxification. When we put good things in, we are replacing the bad things. Eventually this will work. If we choose to try and get rid of the toxic burden we have accumulated at the same time, I believe the process to be optimized. By that, I mean the process for your perfect new healthy lifestyle. Some of the best and most effective ways to detoxify the body are luxurious and relaxing.

Detoxifying—Far Infrared Sauna

My favorite way to detoxify is using a far infrared sauna. Not all saunas are created equal. I have always had low blood pressure which always got me when using saunas. The effect for me in a steam sauna, or even a dry sauna is to feel like a wilted plant or flower. I had no energy once walking out of the sauna and felt completely sapped. I would usually be spent for the day. While in these saunas I often felt like I was unable to breathe, my lungs strained against the steamy air. A far infrared sauna has the opposite effect. If you are like me and could never enjoy the experience of a sauna, then you will need to try this one for yourself to see the difference. A FIR sauna is an incredible tool for your health and used widely in many healing establishments. Far infrared light is the healing powers of the sun. No life can exist without the sun. Plant life needs the sun for photosynthesis. We need the sun for warmth and light. The light from our sun promotes the production of gamma globulin, increases white blood cell count, and enhances the oxygen carrying capacity of our red blood cells. The rays of the sun are varied, some harmful when too exposed to them, and some very nourishing and healing. Sunblock is used to stave off the harmful effects of the UV light which can cause skin cancer if we are exposed to too much. Much of this problem has been exacerbated in recent years due to the deterioration of the ozone layer from our contamination problems on Earth. I am sure there are other hidden reasons that skin cancer has been on the rise, however, we know that these harmful rays from the sun are part of the reason. Far infrared light has been identified as healing in many different ways that affect our lives and it comes from the sun.

When we contract a virus, it runs through our body affecting our cells. Our bodies react by trying to eliminate this unwanted guest by whatever means they can. One of these amazing ways is to create a fever. Our bodies will create an internal heat of at least 102 degrees F. in order to flush out the virus. Our bodies know that at 102 degrees all pathogens die. What the body is trying to do is bring us to the boiling point of the pathogens we are carrying in a valiant attempt at flushing them out. What is the first thing you do when you get a fever? We lower it. We take something—from the modern medicine we all store in the medicine cabinets—that is designed to block this fever reaction leaving us defenseless. Remember when I explained what happens each time we take an aspirin? Acetaminophen and ibuprofen are equally harmful to the body, affecting the liver as well as the stomach lining, just like the aspirin. We cut the legs out from under us when we do this. A fever is only dangerous when it gets to a very high point that might endanger our internal organs. I am not a doctor and I do not intend to contradict any doctor's orders. I am simply trying to explain things that we should all know about health and our bodies. For the purposes of this topic, how to clean out pathogens (and other toxins) from our bodies, using FIR is much the same effect as a fever. FIR light is reproduced inside the sauna and is able to penetrate the skin deeply. The invisible light heats up cells from within and consequently can heat up to 140 degrees or more without damage. Cells that receive too much heat will simply shut down and stop receiving but no damage will result. There are no negative side effects. The only side effects are positive.

When we use a FIR sauna at any temperature at or above 102 degrees, we effectively reduce pathogens from our bodies. How this works is because we store toxins in our fat cells. Not all, but a good majority of the chemical exposure, like from heavy metals, is stored in these fat cells. Those of us with a sedentary lifestyle will be more at risk of toxic overload when these toxins continue to pile up, with no relief in sight. Of all the doctors and PhDs that I have listened to and trained with, all of them concur on this one tool—the FIR sauna is a great defense against the contamination we live with. It is something we can use every day with no negative side effects. The heat is relaxing and the effects are positive. When used every day, we lower our toxicity levels, reducing lead, mercury, nickel, and cadmium which are some of the heavy metals that get stored in our fat cells. We also have the ability to remove alcohol, nicotine, and sulfuric acid through the sweat glands that are stimulated by the far infrared light. My small far infrared sauna is my favorite way to unwind and know that I am doing a great thing for my body. Since the heat increases circulation in the body, it is able to carry off metabolic waste further enhancing the great effects. Muscles get oxygen rich blood delivered and recover faster, and there is the wonderful side effect of weight loss that is virtually effortless. Yes, it is a great weight loss tool as well. An hour in the sauna can be a great way to burn off hundreds of calories. It's a win-win for all.

Detoxifying—Fasting

Delving into the detoxification process further, fasting is a great way to rid the body of unwanted materials. It is also an incredible way to allow the processes in the body other than the digestive tract to get the well-deserved attention from the blood flow.

Fasting is a word that seems to scare many. To fast is simply to delay the act of chewing food for the time one has set apart for the fast. Some cultures of the world fast as a way of religious observance. There is evidence, as with many of the older traditions found, that fasting provided a way to stay healthy in a time when there were no hospitals or doctors for that matter. People had to fight the diseases of the times with whatever means they had and many cultures survived simply due to good, and often clean-living habits. When we eat food, chewing it as much as possible is key as it aids the stomach in the process of breaking it down. The stomach has to work less if we chew our food properly. Saliva is also a precursor to the digestion of food and helps also to properly digest it. When we fast for our health the idea is to get your nutrition for the day in liquid form. If we are drinking our meals for a 24-hour period for example, we actively help our digestive process to take a rest. The process of distributing nutrition from liquid is decidedly less taxing than digesting chewable food. The other factor that is so helpful is allowing the other processes in the body to receive the attention of our circulatory flow in order for them to be allowed to recover and regenerate. We have so many systems in the body, running all the time to keep us alive and well. We have the circulatory system, lymphatic, respiratory, excretory, and the nervous system to name a few.

When we eat, our cells realize that the job is to digest and distribute our nutrition. If we spend a day as we usually do, by eating at least three meals a day, we are basically using our digestive system constantly. When we fast for a day, or any length of time, our digestive tract is not the star of the show anymore and the other processes are using their time wisely. We allow for recovery and regeneration, a general clean up if you will. Fasting can be used in many different ways and is easily incorporated to our unique lifestyles. I know those that prefer a 24-hour fast every week for the effect that it has on their energy and clarity. I also know those that prefer an intermittent fasting schedule as it is better suited to them. A popular way of intermittent fasting is to skip breakfast and restrict your eating periods to 8 hours a day. The 16 hours left in the 24-hour period is the fasting period. It is not very painful and I have been doing it for the past 8 years almost. The energy that is produced in my body by giving it a rest from the act of eating is crazy. I always achieve a clarity that I have come to rely on. I enjoy good food but I also enjoy everything much more when I feel great and have clarity of thought as much as possible. There is an element of discipline we add to our lives when we engage in these cleansing strategies. We become more thoughtful of what we are doing when we do things with purpose. Your body has done so much for you, isn't it time you treated it like the amazing temple that it truly is?

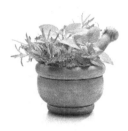

Chapter 8

Healing Through Science and Technology

There exists today a huge market of extremely effective, science-based alternative modalities of healing. Technology is also advancing in ways that can help us to find non-invasive, new therapies to heal just about everything. The same advancement that is affecting our environment for the worse, in many ways, is also giving us incredible tools for healing which we haven't seen before.

Each healer that I have studied has chosen one avenue of healing for the body. If you were to look at which of our organs are more useful to us you would find that it's hard to determine because they all work together in a synergistic way. This is why each healer has a unique way of looking at the body. Each healer has a chosen area of expertise. The body is an incredibly complex network of life. To narrow the focus to get to a part you understand better than another, something that resonates with you more than any other thing, then becomes your focus. The instruments of healing that I will introduce to you represent this idea. Some have stumbled upon these truths and others have actually invented ways to help the body do what it was meant to do, only with a little help from science. New problems require new ways of thinking to solve them. Granted, these ideas are not all actually new, but the ways that have been found by these inventors and healers to put old ideas to use with new technology is no less than amazing.

The first instrument uses the constant source of natural healing energy, the earth. I am talking about Earthing, or as some call it, Grounding. Let's back track for a moment and define electrons. Google dictionary defines an electron as "A stable subatomic particle with a charge of negative electricity, found in all atoms and acting as the primary carrier of electricity in solids." We need voltage for our bodies to work properly. We need electrons to heal. And because electrons have a negative charge, that makes it a donor, meaning it gives energy or electricity. If something has a positive charge, it will be an electron stealer. This simply means that something with a positive charge will be looking to bond with your electrons and tap your energy. The opposite is what we want to focus on. We want to know as many ways as possible to get more electrons to our bodies, that add energy and help us heal.

Growing up, I did not really get the whole idea of chemistry. I did well in the class, but I hardly remember the ideas I learned. Now I find chemistry a fascinating subject. So much of life as I see it now is chemistry. Another fascinating subject that escaped me as a young student was electrical engineering. The idea of electrical engineering has taken on a completely new meaning for me today.

Grounding

We have free-flowing electrons at our disposal. The ground under us is exactly this. Our Earth is a constant source of this healing energy. It is abundant with electrons that flow through the ground to your feet and up to where your body might need it most. Any natural contact with the earth restores your body's natural electrical state because we live on an electrical planet. When we walk barefoot on the natural soil we are able to absorb the electrons the earth freely gives. The most obvious benefits to this are reduced pain, reduced stress, and reduced inflammation. Inflammation is one of the world's worst stresses of our bodies and consequently, life. It is known to cause premature aging as well as chronic pain and stress. Inflammation is one way our bodies deal with a problem. We send blood to the area in question in an attempt to get more nutrients to heal, but when we have not put enough nutrients in our bodies we can use, we create a chronic condition, inflammation. We can't always see this inflammation, but we can certainly feel it. Grounding ourselves is one answer that definitely works.

If you know an electrical engineer, you can ask them to explain why we need grounding wires in our houses. In electronic circuit theory, a "ground" is an infinite source for charge, something that can absorb an unlimited amount of current without changing its potential. A common return path for current. The ground is an unlimited potential. When we walk barefoot, we absorb an endless flow of electrons that will heal us, by grounding us, and balancing our energy. This only happens with direct contact with the earth. Another source for unlimited natural electrons is the ocean. A dynamic body of water is an electron donor. A still body of water is not an electron donor. Those of us that live by the ocean can understand how healthy this can be if we take advantage of it. All of us have the option of taking off our shoes and standing on the ground near us. The very smart folks that have thought of a great way to make these powers of healing more accessible to us have come up with amazing grounding tools for use inside. A grounding blanket and/or sheets made with silver wire in the fabric is an excellent substitute and you can absorb the energy for the length of time you are sleeping. I have had one for approximately eight years. I also live close to the sea. I love walking on the sand by the ocean with my feet in the water as much as I can. I do not suffer from inflammation. I have been a martial artist for almost twenty years and I have old injuries. I have been told by a sports surgeon that I have rheumatoid arthritis in my body, but still have yet to suffer any pain or inflammation. There are a few other products made for specific jobs that may cause stress or inflammation, such as working on the computer, or a hairdresser for example. Those that sit for a long time while at work can use a mat that will ground them where they work. Same concept for those that are standing in one place, mats that can ground you while you work for the hairdresser for example. The evidence is there. The science is sound. This energy can be measured. There are those that believe the invention of the shoe has been one of the reasons we now suffer from so many autoimmune diseases and inflammation. Shoes have cut us off from our natural source of healing we once enjoyed a long time ago. I always say, this is not about whether you believe it or not, science clearly backs it up. It is only whether or not you decide to see for yourself.

The Circulatory System

We have an amazing system of transport within our bodies that is practically unparalleled. Our powerful heart pumps blood through the main arteries, but we have an incredible amount of microvessels that carry blood to every remote part of our body. We have something approximate to 74,000 miles of capillaries in our bodies that aid in transporting nutrients, hormones, basically everything to our entire body. These microvessels also help cleanse our blood, taking waste to where it needs to go as it flows through. As we all know, our blood flow should never be restricted or impeded in any way. Unless of course we are badly wounded and losing blood. This is not the scenario we are working with. When we eat too much trans fats, we may do some damage to our arteries. Literally, it is our diet that will affect what happens to our arteries and our blood flow. Exercise is an incredibly helpful tool, but we will tackle that one later. In any case, we are all approaching this from different angles as we are all at different stages in our lives. Different ages, different backgrounds, etc. This is what drew me to a product called the BEMER, the Bio Electric Magnetic Energy Regulator. It is effective. No matter our circumstance, the BEMER works. If heart disease is one of the leading causes of death in the U.S., then it's a no brainer that something that will help your blood circulate better, no matter what your habits have been, is vital. The BEMER works with a technology that uses a wave that stimulates vasomotion. In fact, this word (and action) was discovered in the 70s. The scientist realized that this wave stimulated the sides of blood vessels to move the blood in the body with better circulation. There is a common misconception that the heart is solely responsible for pumping the blood everywhere. This would be quite a job for our heart. Despite being a very strong muscle, our heart couldn't possibly do all the work alone. It is the vessels that respond with the action called vasomotion that picks up any slack. The BEMER was discovered to stimulate this particular motion with an amazing effect on the body. Since we know that we need nutrition for our blood to be able to nourish our entire bodies from within, then it really stands to reason that better blood flow would carry the nourishment faster than it could travel otherwise. The faster the travel, the faster the healing. The premise is faster circulation, faster healing. Our circulation can be improved upon in more than one way.

Exercise is a very important factor for our health. I have learned over the year in my business that no one can be forced to enjoy exercise. My mother was a very sedentary person. She enjoyed stillness and peace. It was her way. My mother was raised in a time when women didn't sweat, and they were always ladylike. She also never had a weight problem therefore exercise was seen by her as useless. This is why I believe a product like the BEMER can help so many people to improve their health. I do not think there are substitutes for hard work put in to our own health, but I do think finding alternative ways to incorporate something we don't always like is important. There are other healing waves out there that work and I have tried them. The one that is most user friendly with the most noticeable effect is the BEMER. I am careful not to endorse any one salvation over another, but finding ways to help those that otherwise would not see a way to accomplish their health goals is what I love to do. If I told you that you could improve your general blood flow, improve your oxygen supply, and waste disposal, cardiac function, physical fitness, endurance, energy, stress reduction, by just laying on a blanket for a few minutes, would you want to know about it? Wherever we are now in our health, whether we are recovering from a stroke, or enduring an autoimmune disease, our metabolic process can be vastly improved by strengthening our circulatory system with some help from these technological advancements in health.

As a health educator and lifestyle consultant, I have no affiliations with any products. I recommend according to the needs of the person educating me about their lives and desires. Free will and some education is key to making decisions about how we want to feel and for how long. There is always a way. When we know better, we must strive to do better. Ideally the BEMER shows us the many rewards to living an active life. We were meant to move. Circulation is part of what keeps us alive and well. We are in a position to accept as much help as we can to not just survive, but thrive in today's world. Tapping into the energy around us, trying to understand what we can't see but know is there, keeps us in touch with unlimited possibilities. I encourage everyone to look things up, information accessibility is instant. See for yourselves what is out there. Look into the science. What resonates with each one of us is what may become a possibility for healing and a new way of life that will enable us to deal with our own personal health once and for all.

Nutritional Showers

As I continued my search for information and healing opportunities, I discovered a company bringing to life a concept that is truly cutting edge and so obvious that I wondered why I never thought of it before: Nutritional showers. We read about the skin as one of the most overlooked organs we have, it is also the largest. Our skin absorbs everything we put on our bodies. That is quite a load. Take one of the products you currently have in your bathroom and read the ingredients. We are organic beings, not made to continuously absorb chemicals and artificial ingredients. Today we barely recognize how many packaged products we use daily. In some households, the more the better. There are lipsticks available on the market today advertised for their lasting power. They contain lead. These large companies have enough money behind them to target their market audience directly. The target audience for makeup products is teenage girls. I have two teenage daughters and it's a constant battle. The older we get the more we understand the effects of how we have or haven't taken care of our own skin. Inside and out. There are several brands all over the world that are using all-natural ingredients for products like shampoo, conditioner, and soap. Lotions are now being replaced with oils. We must pay attention to the warnings we hear about different ingredients as they do penetrate the skin and enter our bodies contributing to the toxic overload. What if I were to tell you, instead of taking medicine, the future equivalent of a doctor would one day be able to prescribe a particular ingredient/herb to be used every day in your shower. If our skin absorbs everything we put on it, then it is also possible to put nutrients into our bodies through the skin. These nutrients would not have to pass through the digestive system, they would permeate the skin quickly, reaching their mark with less process. Our bodies were meant to have at least seventy-four plus minerals and metals as nutrients once abundant in our environment. We are suffering collectively from deficiencies, and toxic overload, and developing chronic conditions as a result. It is becoming harder and harder to learn the best nutritional choices we have, let alone find them from a reliable source.

I have met the owner/inventor of this nutritional shower and I have seen its effectiveness personally. Using a dark field microscope to see the blood before and after showed my blood cells to behave differently. My blood was sticky and slightly sluggish before my shower. After a ten-minute shower with this magical water my blood was glowing. It was no longer sticky and each cell had a glow around it. Even my white blood cells had more mobility than before. The idea is amazing and the reality even more. Most of these products are not cheap. What does not cost us, we do not value. The concept of this shower is to put into our bodies the nutrients, i.e., ionized minerals that we all need, through water. The shower boasts the cleanest water possible, using the highest standards of filtration and structuring, then adding raw materials we call humic/fulvic minerals that our bodies need that we no longer find easily. Fulvic comes from original, plant-based material. Humic is a plant source based liquid solution with all the trace minerals found naturally in organic plant materials. This is added to the stream of water. The temperature of the water is hot so it will drive the nutrients into the body through our open pores. This starts a process of healing in the blood that is actually visible when seen through a dark field. This is a wide-open field that few have heard of as the technology is so specific. Not too many people know of its existence. Those that do know of it, have done everything in their power to either own one, or have access to one. There are studies being done in different parts of the country to measure the effects of the nutritious water on illnesses like diabetes, ALS, and so many more. The process is patent pending. The delivery system of the water is unique and has to do with the molecular structure. There is absolutely nothing that can do any harm. Only good. These showers will become commercially available and will be more affordable in a few years. They are currently on the market and are very expensive. How much is your health worth to you?

Light Energy and Frequencies
There are a few other methods of healing that are coming out into the world and showing us how we haven't really begun to investigate the different ways we all can heal. The

subject of biophotonic light/energy is also a fascinating idea. Each one of these healing devices is non-invasive, and simple. Each one can be incorporated into everyone's daily life. Biophotonic treatment consists of using a visible red or near infra light energy to encourage our cells to do several different things. The process puts into action gene transcription and also cellular repair, among other magical reactions that are incredible for the body. There are small units that put out the biophotonic light we can use to treat our blood. One that I have used is a small bulb that attaches to a nostril with the bulb inside. As the blood passes through our entire body it will pass through this one spot approximately every twenty minutes. The membranes in our noses are thin enough for the light to affect the blood without having to invade the body with surgery or needles.

Frequencies are now extremely interesting when used for healing. Everything in our bodies has a frequency. Every organ has its basic frequency that when thrown off creates problems. Remember our bodies are constantly seeking balance. The healing part is when we are able to find the same or similar frequency in nature, we can reprogram our own system by matching it. Smell is one way for us to be affected by frequency. That is exactly what aromatherapy is. A healthy body ranges from about 62-80 HZ. When our body drops lower than 50 HZ, we are in trouble. This is just another approach to seeing how to reach a balance again in the body when it feels off. In nature, there are frequencies that can help us by raising our own frequency or vibration to match the one around us. This can be accomplished by simply smelling it, or being near its light as we see in biophotonic modulation. Do your due diligence on any product that claims too much. Always ask about the science behind what they are selling. Talk with the owners if you can. It is very important to be safe and not do anything that could cause any harm.

All of the amazing technologies I've mentioned here have an interaction (in the form of improvement and healing) with different parts of the body. They should not be considered cures, or even replacements for the work that needs to take place in each of us. We are the ones that need to change the way we eat. We are the ones that know exercise is really important. We know drinking water is very important. When we learn to define why these things are important and how our bodies react to them, we can start to visualize our way to healing. When we can understand what is happening in our own bodies we can learn to listen better and be more in tune with what we need at any given time.

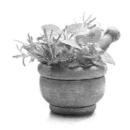

Chapter 9

Move into Your Health and Happiness

The subject of exercise is so controversial in the sense that it means different things to different people. Americans are divided in the area of athletics. Americans revere the athlete on the highest level, but resent their neighbor for being in great shape because they work out all the time. A professional athlete is one of the highest paid careers in the world. We all sit spellbound and exhilarated when watching our favorite events in the Olympic Games every four years. An Olympic athlete is the representation of the power and magnificence of the human body. They become the ultimate expression of the human spirit through their steadfast discipline. In Ancient Greek times, the Olympians came to represent not only physical strength but also spiritual strength. The code of ethics and morality associated with the athlete was held in the highest esteem. After all, a person dedicated to the transcendence of physical and mental limits must be driven by higher ideals. The manifestation of a perfect body and incredible physical skill comes through the strongest willpower and strength of spirit. We encourage our children to be active, to play sports, and we tell them they will grow up strong. What happens after that? We become too busy? We are busy with "more important" ideas and needs? We make a decision to leave sports to the athletes, giving up our sneakers for car keys. We forget the natural needs of our bodies to be in motion, hiding behind our very busy schedules. The truth is there is always time for the things we want to do. What you feed grows and what you starve dies, is the old adage. If we see sports or exercise as something for other people, then it will be. If you are able to find a physical activity that you enjoy, you will do it more often. If you do it more often, you will see the results and be reinforced to continue. A friend of mine is married to a woman with a terrible work schedule. She never had time for anything until they took a rescue dog into their home. This woman was so in love with her new four-legged companion that she would get up at 5 a.m. to walk the dog before leaving for work. At night, again she would walk her beloved pet before hitting the hay. Her husband, my friend, was amazed and very happy to have noticed that his wife's figure had regained some shape, and he was over the moon at how attractive she had become to him again. They have been married for over thirty years. The lesson here is that just walking down the street and back, twice a day, was enough to have had an effect on her physical shape.

I know of one unspoken rule that never wavers: exercise without a good diet will not bring the results we want, and dieting without exercise won't either. We might succeed in changing something, but it will not last. Maybe if we eliminated the word exercise, we would not be affected by the idea of it, enabling us to be more wanton with the possibilities that physical fitness could give us. Any movement that is balanced, and something we do every day, is good for us. That is it. It doesn't have to be a hockey league, or a gym membership, God forbid. Movement is so diverse and varied that the options are almost unlimited. I will give some excellent examples in this chapter of all the interesting things I have tried and chosen, and why. They are only examples. If you live close to the sea, a walk by the ocean every day would be spectacular. Even if you are there for twenty or fifteen minutes. Koreans are surrounded by many mountains and hills, giving them their favorite past time as a culture, hiking.

There is a difference in exercise as we get older, and our bodies change. As young people we think about muscles and being strong. When we form muscles, we are making energy. Muscles are basically a battery that provides us with extra energy. This is how our bodies reinforce that exercise/ movement is needed. As we get older muscles become a thing of the past. The good news for us older folk is we don't need to do grinding workouts anymore. We realize that the most important thing is our fascia. Fascia is the thin sheath of fibrous tissue that encloses muscles and organs. Fascia is responsible for attaching everything that needs to be attached to your body. Imagine a sheet of connective tissue all of your body, keeping everything where it should be. This sounds way more important than a big muscle doesn't it? When we are young, we want what looks good. As we age, we realize that we look good if we can keep everything in its place. The exercise needed to grow a muscle is very specific. It is a matter of breaking down the muscle for it to heal and grow from the scar tissue. This is only temporary unless you decide to keep up the strength training forever. What we need to strengthen our fascia is less arduous but equally, if not more, important. Remember the story of the tortoise and the hare? Slow and steady wins the race. The same is true in this case. It is not about how much weight you can lift, it is more a question of form. We must learn to keep our fascia strong and healthy to keep our vitality and health throughout our body.

Weight bearing exercise is most important for our bones as we get older. All the research still shows how important weight bearing exercise still is for the body. We know this from the problems of osteoporosis. The old saying "use it or lose it" holds true. If we don't use our strength, we tend to lose it slowly. Same with range of mobility. Nutrition is also vital if we expect our fascia to continue holding us together. In fact, cellulite only shows when we have maligned and unhealthy fascia. There is great evidence that is showing older generations don't need such a strenuous workout anymore. Most beneficial to strength, balance, weight, and overall looks is simply a core exercise program that lasts about fifteen minutes a day. There are many things we can do to incorporate these fifteen minutes that we can devote just to ourselves every day. Some suggestions I have are yoga, for example. There are so many programs on TV or online that will give us a nice, complete yoga routine that we can follow along with daily. I have something called a rebounder at home that I love. This rebounder is like a small round mini trampoline. It fits almost anywhere indoors. The idea is to bounce on it for about fifteen minutes a day. Do this and you will feel a difference. A rebounder not only strengthens your legs and core, but it also provides a kind of exercise for the cells. The gravitational pull on the cells themselves provides a pulling and reshaping of the circle of our cells. This has a hand in keeping our cells active and resilient. Besides all that, it is actually fun.

I will confess I have always been an athlete. Growing up I was a tomboy. I had no looks to speak of so I was not distracted from my pursuit of MVP or any championships for teams I played on. I always loved sports. I was naturally very good at them. Any sport was my favorite. I even played basketball for my college in Germany while I was there. I never had a problem with exercise. Growing up, sports was the answer to many things for me. After I had my second daughter at thirty-four, my options were limited. I knew I needed to get back to some kind of physical activity but I didn't know what. I have never been in love with running just to run, my second confession. I joined a gym. I had lots of classes to choose from at the gym. This was how I was first introduced to martial arts. I started with a kick box cardio class at the gym. I literally felt like Bruce Lee after a few weeks. I realized I was very good at it and also loved it enormously. I felt so empowered every time I left the gym. Soon I realized that my training at the gym was limited and I did some research on a karate class in the area. This was my new sport. I have trained for over ten years in several different forms of martial arts since then and I highly recommend this. There is no ceiling to the learning in a traditional martial arts class. It is very important to find a class that suits you and does not force any of its students to do things they are not prepared to do. The reason why so many injuries happen is because of the ego. This is a danger in any gym, dojo, or anywhere there are athletes. We need to keep that ego in check. There is no need to break a wooden board unless it is something you are intent on doing for your own reasons. Competition is no longer useful. The only competing we should do is with ourselves. I am also not keen on fighting for sport. I love the discipline and poetry of traditional karate. I love the history and the magic of the movements. I love the speed and agility it gives me. I love the incredible workout it gives me, body, and mind. The trick is to find something you like to do. How do we know we like something if we haven't tried it? We don't! We must try things in order to find what puts a smile on our face and gives us peace of mind that we are doing good things for our bodies. If we feel good, we keep doing what is good for us. If you are a loner, do something you can do solo. Take a walk every day. Take a gym class you like. Go for a swim. If you don't know how to swim, take classes. I can't stress enough the importance of physical activity to heal a body. Take heed and your body will thank you.

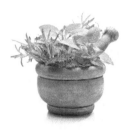

Chapter 10

The Healing Crisis

The healing crisis refers to how we feel when we begin to change our diets and lifestyles for the better. As we detoxify, it can be a devastating reaction for some of us. There is often a period of time that we feel bad, even sick. This is a reaction to changing things from bad, to good. Any change takes some getting used to. If we quit doing what we are doing because it feels different or perhaps not as good, we might jeopardize our healing process. The trick is to take it slowly. Do your research and be sure of what you are doing. When we detoxify too quickly our bodies may suffer. If this happens, simply slow down and reduce the stress to the changes. Your body will love you, if you give it a chance to do what it naturally wants to do—and that is to be perfect.

There is so much new science in our world today that we need a guide to help us find the answers that pertain to us. When my parents became ill, I spent all my time studying everything health related that I could get my hands on. I had never been touched by death or illness until then. Somehow I knew that my future depended on my research. I had two small children by that time. I knew the fate of my grandparents on either side, each having either cancer or heart disease. I did not want to believe as most do, that I was doomed to this fate as well. I also couldn't accept this fate for my children. I knew that I had to change my life and world. It was already changing, I just had to steer it better. Genetic history is only a part of our cellular identity. Where we come from is in our genes, but where we are going, only we decide. We do not have to follow the same path. The science I have learned has taught me that genes can be turned on and they can also be turned off. It is like flipping a switch. We have the switches inside, we are born with them. It is our free will that gives us the choice to live with it, or to change it.

I use the switch metaphor because sometimes it is as easy flipping a switch to turn a light on or off. Let's say we have the indicated gene for developing lung cancer, would you smoke? This would be an indication of turning on the genetic code for developing lung cancer. If you already smoked, the best result would be for you to decide to quit. This would be your best bet for turning off that switch. Quitting smoking is one of the hardest things to do, but it is basically a decision you make. You would know that this is the right answer. The next steps would be to find help in accomplishing this task. Anything we can find to help us, reinforce us, support us, these are the things that help us succeed. Taking the decision into your own hands is the most empowering thing in the world. I urge you to take your health seriously. Taking steps to find what is the best way to prevent illness, and strengthen the immune system, is far better than fighting your way back to health. If you have worked your whole life to succeed in business, to provide well for your family, then health is your next project. It is not easy in our world to keep our health when we are constantly being bombarded with pollution, contaminants, and the by-product of more and more profit. Even our food has changed. Nutrition is no longer at the forefront. Don't wait for the ball to drop. Don't be afraid to create a lifestyle change. If the change is initiated by you for good reasons, then the experience can be exciting. Knowledge is power. When I meet a friend that warns me, "Don't get too close, I have a cold!" I always laugh and tell them not to worry, I am impervious! The reality is that I haven't suffered a cold in over five years. The people I have helped also tell me they have not had so much as a cold since changing their health lifestyle. My purpose is to educate. The doctors I work with always say they can make someone better, but only you can decide if you want to stay well. As my trainer used to tell me, 90% you, 10% trainer. With the right view and education, I can enable my readers and clients to deal with their own personal health. We should all question whether or not we are using nutrition to be healthier, to avoid DNA damage. Or are we just putting things into our mouths without thinking of the effect it might have on us later. What you feed grows, what you starve dies. If you have learned one new thing from my information you didn't know before, then I am successful. There is so much incredible new technology today to help us create a new health lifestyle, are you taking advantage of it? The research I have done, is the research you don't have to do. When our bodies are clear, our minds are also clear. We have come to this life with one body, it is only fitting that we take care of it as it is our only instrument here on Earth. My goal is to educate as many people as I can to understand that there is no higher organization that cares about your health as much as you care. There is no governmental organization that is morally bound to make sure all of your food and water is void of toxins.

Acknowledgements

I would like to thank my daughters for their love and support during this time for me. Without their constant support I would not have been able to finish my book. Especially to my daughter Asia. She is now a spirit guide watching over her family. I am forever grateful for the chance to have been her mother for the 20 years she blessed us with her loving company.

To Dr. Jerry Tennant, the fabulous physician that you are. I've learned so much from you. Thank you.

To Leo Symborski, thank you for all that you do to keep all of us healthy and happy.

To the Morgan James Publishing team: Special thanks to David Hancock, CEO & Founder for believing in me and my message. To my Author Relations Manager, Margo Toulouse, thanks for making the process seamless and easy. Many more thanks to everyone else, but especially Jim Howard, Bethany Marshall, and Nickcole Watkins.

Thank You

Thank you for allowing me to guide you on this informational journey to health. I am truly grateful for the trust you have placed in me and I hope that I have given you some things to think about. If you have learned one thing that you didn't know before, then I have been successful. I understand there is a lot of information in this book and that is why I have created my companion program for one-on-one strategy sessions and accountability measures to further guide you to your perfect health lifestyle.

If you and your team would like to work with me to achieve greater health, feel free to reach out and schedule a strategy session with me. If you are interested in a full immersion, educational health retreat in a gorgeous, exotic location where only your health will be the focus, simply email me at karatefitness@att.net.

About the Author

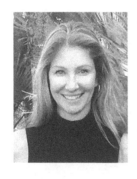

Maria Teresa Kline is a very open-minded individual with unique perspectives on life. Speaking over four languages, she has spent most of her life immersed in cultures around the world. Born in Africa to an American diplomat, Maria Teresa moved to a new place almost every two years of her life. Maria has lived in many countries around the world, on five of the seven continents. She is well traveled to say the least. Attending several universities around the world, Maria graduated with a degree in political science, a minor in both philosophy and psychology. A natural teacher,

Maria taught English in several countries, including South Korea and Costa Rica, but decided to pursue a different avenue of teaching when she settled in Florida to raise her two beautiful daughters. She trained in the martial arts and became a karate instructor. It was during this time that Maria's father was diagnosed with a rare brain degenerative disease, and her mother with breast cancer shortly thereafter. In light of this, Maria dedicated herself to learning and later teaching others about health. Pursuing this she became a certified health educator from Hippocrates Health Institute, a certified raw vegan chef, and a certified life coach. She has since spent her life devoted to helping others master health and better themselves physically, spiritually, and emotionally. Maria has spent years cultivating her knowledge on the human body and what should go into it. She is also well versed in iridology, the study of irises, a noninvasive way to indicate illness. A reformed meat eater Maria has been vegan for over seven years now. Maria feels strongly about sharing her extensive and diverse knowledge and is doing so by publishing a nationwide attainable book with simple, easy-to-follow guidelines for achieving great health.